The Vibrant Guide to Plant-Based Desserts

Easy and Tasty Dessert Recipes to Start Your Plant-Based Diet and Boost Your Lifestyle

Clay Palmer

Table of Contents

Fragrant Spiced Coffee

Servings: 8 Preparation time: 2 hours and 10 minutes

Ingredients:

4 cinnamon sticks, each about 3 inches long 1 1/2 teaspoons of whole cloves 1/3 cup of honey 2-ounce of chocolate syrup 1/2 teaspoon of anise extract 8 cups of brewed coffee

Directions:

Pour the coffee in a 4-quarts slow cooker and pour in the remaining ingredients except for cinnamon and stir properly. Wrap the whole cloves in cheesecloth and tie its corners with strings. Immerse this cheesecloth bag in the liquid present in the slow cooker and cover it with the lid. Then plug in the slow cooker and let it cook on the low heat setting for 3 hours or until heated thoroughly. When done, discard the cheesecloth bag and serve.

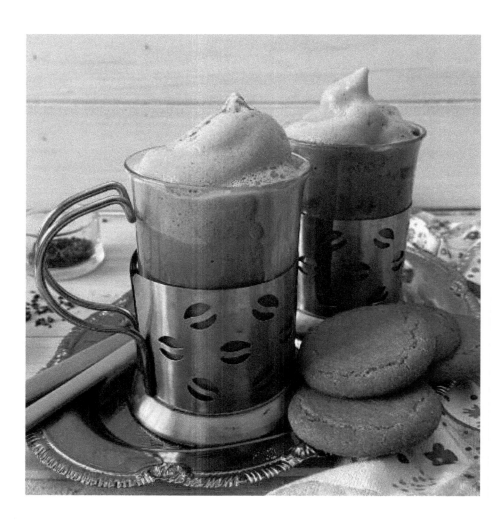

Apple Pudding

Preparation time: 5 minutesCooking time: 30 minutes
Servings: 2

Ingredients:

3 large pippin (tart green) apples 4 Tbs. butter 3 Tbs.
sugar ½ tsp. cinnamon ¼ tsp. ground cloves 1 tsp.
grated lemon rind batter 3 eggs ½ cup flour 1½ cups milk
3 Tbs. sugar 2 Tbs. brandy ½ tsp. vanilla extract dash
of nutmeg garnish ¼ to ½ cup confectioners' sugar

Directions:

Quarter, peel, and core the apples and cut the quarters
in thin slices. In a shallow, fireproof casserole, sauté the
apple slices in butter for several minutes. Add the sugar,
cinnamon, cloves, and lemon rind and continue to cook
the apples, stirring often, for another 5 minutes, or until
the apples are just tender. Beat together the eggs, flour,
milk, sugar, brandy, vanilla, and nutmeg, or blend them
in a blender. Pour the batter over the apples and bake
the pudding for 25 to 30 minutes ina preheated oven at
400 degrees, or until it is puffed and golden brown on
top. Sift confectioners' sugar over the top of the pudding
and serve it warm with coffee or milk.

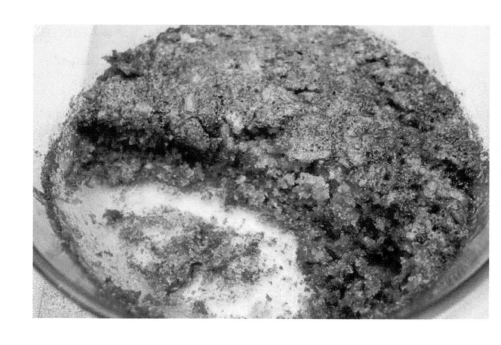

Fruit Torte

Preparation time: 5 minutesCooking time: 45 minutes

Servings: 2

Ingredients:

6 tablespoons (98 g) unsalted butter, at room temperature, plus 1/3 cup sugar 2 large eggs, separated 1 cup unbleached almond flour 2 ½ teaspoons baking powder ¼ cup heavy cream 2 teaspoons almond extract 2 ripe plums, apricots, or nectarines, sliced 1 cup blueberries Confectioners' sugar, for dusting

Directions: Preheat the oven to 350°F (180°C). Butter a 9-inch (23 cm) tart pan with a removable bottom. Add a round of parchment, butter the parchment, then flour it. Place 6 tablespoons (84 g) of butter and 1/3 cup (67 g) sugar in the bowl of an electric mixer fitted with the paddle attachment. Beat together on low speed until smooth and fluffy. Add the egg yolks and beat well until combined. In a small bowl, stir together the flour and the baking powder. In another small bowl, stir together the cream, ¼ cup (60 ml) water, anise or almond extract, and vanilla extract. Stir the mixtures into the butter mixture by alternating the flour mixture with the cream mixture—adding one-third of each at a time until they are used up. In a clean bowl fitted to an electric mixer using a whisk attachment, whip the egg whites until stiff peaks form. If the eggs are not stiff enough, the cake will not rise properly. Using a rubber spatula, gently fold the beaten egg whites into the batter to eliminate all of the white and break up any lumps. Then stir once in the opposite direction to make sure that all white has been incorporated. Pour the batter into the prepared tart pan and level the surface. Arrange the plums or other fruit in a circle pattern on top of the batter. Sprinkle the remaining tablespoon (13 g) of sugar on top of the fruit. Bake until a toothpick inserted into the middle of the cake comes out clean and cake begins to pull away from the sides of the pan, 35 to 40 minutes. Transfer to a cooling rack. Allow cake to cool for at least 30 minutes. Invert onto a cooling rack and remove sides of pan, then bottom and parchment paper. Turn over to cool completely. Invert the cake onto another plate and then back over onto a serving platter. Dust with confectioners' sugar. Serve at room temperature.

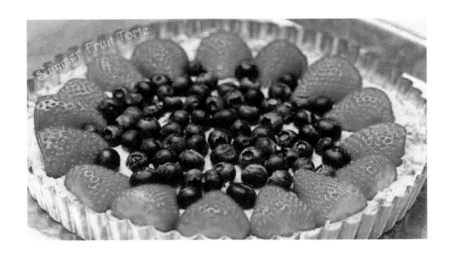

Strawberry Crepes

Preparation time: 5 minutesCooking time: 35 minutes
Servings: 2

Ingredients:

Crepe batter: 2 eggs ½ cup all-purpose flour 1 tbsp. sugar 1 cup milk 1 ½ cups water 2 tbsp. olive oil Filling: 3 cups fresh, sliced strawberries 1 cup granulated sugar ½ cup cottage cheese 1 cup sour cream ½ cup powdered sugar

Directions:

Beat eggs in a bowl. Add a little bit of the flour and sugar. Use an electric mixer or whisk to combine. Then add a little bit of the milk and water. Mix. Repeat the same procedure until all milk, flour, sugar, and water are added. whisk the mixture until a smooth consistency is achieved. Beat in melted butter. Chill batter at least 1 hour. In the meantime, combine strawberries and granulated sugar. Set aside. Beat cottage cheese in a blender or with an electric mixer until smooth. Add sour cream and powdered sugar and stir well. When batter is chilled, heat a crepe pan on medium-high heat. Pour batter into the pan. Swirl batter to coat the entire bottom of the pan and cook for about 2 minutes, or until the bottom of the crepe is firm. Use a fork to gently lift crepe from pan. Flip crepe over. Cook for another minute, or until crepe just starts to brown. Remove to a plate and repeat with remaining Use about µ of fruit and creamy mixture to fill crepes. Fold crepes over. Garnish with powdered sugar.

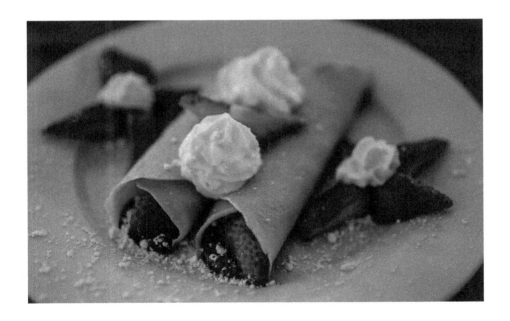

Vegan Strawberry Pie

Preparation time: 15 minutes Cooking time: 45 minutes 6 Slices.

Ingredients:

¾ cup raw cashews 1 cup oats 12 pitted and diced dates 4 tbsp. apple juice 3 tbsp. lemon juice 1 package firm silken tofu 1 tsp. grated lemon rind 1 ½ tbsp.. ground chia seeds 1 tsp. vanilla 2 tsp. agar powder 10 ounces sliced strawberries

Directions:

Begin by placing the cashews in some water and allowing them to soak for one hour. Afterwards, place six dates in a food processor along with some oats. Next, add 2 tbsp. of your apple juice to the processor. This creates a sticky consistency. Press this creation into the bottom of your pie pan. Next, add the cashews to the blender along with the rest of the dates, the tofu, the lemon juice, the chia seeds, the lemon rind, and the vanilla. Blend the ingredients until they're smooth. To the side, heat apple juice and agar powder. Stir and heat the mixture until it begins to boil. Pour this juice into the blender and blend on high. Next, pour this mixture over the piecrust, and allow the pie to chill for three hours in the refrigerator.

Cover the top of the pie with sliced strawberries and enjoy.

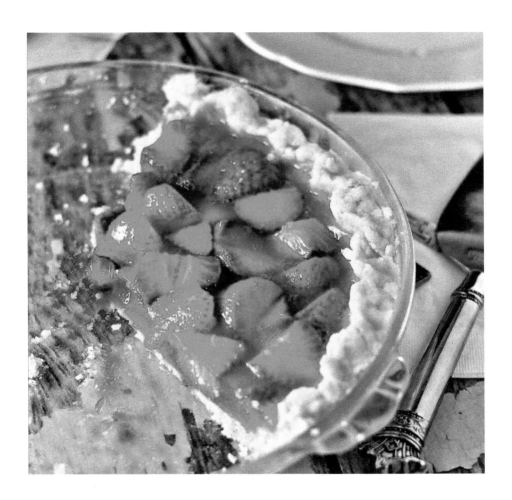

Vegan Chocolate Cake

Preparation time: 15 minutes Cooking time: 35 minutes 1 Cake.

Ingredients:

2 cups all-purpose flour 1 cup sugar 1 tsp. baking soda 1 tsp. salt ½ cup cocao powder 1/3 cup canola oil 2 tsp. vanilla 1 tsp. white vinegar 1 ½ cups chilled water Chocolate Frosting Ingredients: 5 ounces instant pudding mix 1 cup almond milk 10 ounces of vegan cool whip

Directions:

Begin by preheating the oven to 350 degrees Fahrenheit. Next, mix together all the dry ingredients from the first ingredient list. Create a hole in the middle of the mixture and pour the wet ingredients into the hole, one by one. Stir the mixture, leaving a few lumps as you go. Next, pour this batter into a cake pan and bake the cake for thirty minutes. After the cake cools, prepare the pudding frosting by mixing together the cool whip, the pudding mix, and the almond milk. Stir well, and spread the frosting over the cooled cake. Serve, and enjoy!

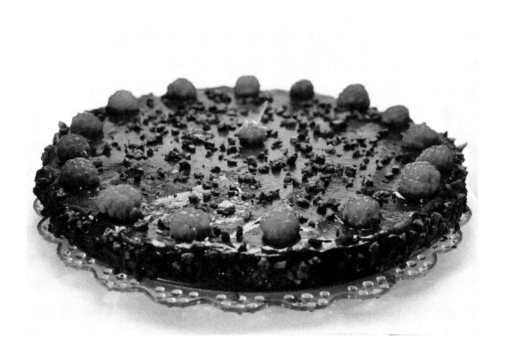

Good Morning Protein Pancakes

Preparation time: 15 minutes Cooking time: 35 minutes 12 vegan pancakes.

Ingredients:

4 cups almond milk 3 tbsp. flax meal 1 tsp. vanilla 2 tsp. apple cider vinegar 3 cups all-purpose flour 1 cup hump protein powder 3 tbsp. sugar 1 tsp. baking powder ½ tsp. baking soda 1 tsp. salt 1 tsp. cinnamon ½ cup canoa oil ½ tsp. ginger

Directions:

Begin by stirring together the almond milk, the flax meal, the vanilla, and the apple cider vinegar. Allow this to sit for ten minutes. Next, mix together all the dry ingredients. After the first mixture has curdled, add the canola oil to it, and bring the wet and dry ingredients together. Stir well. Next, prepare a skillet with a bit of oil, and portion out about a fourth cup of batter out onto the skillet. Cook one side for about three minutes and then flip to cook the other side. Enjoy your pancakes!

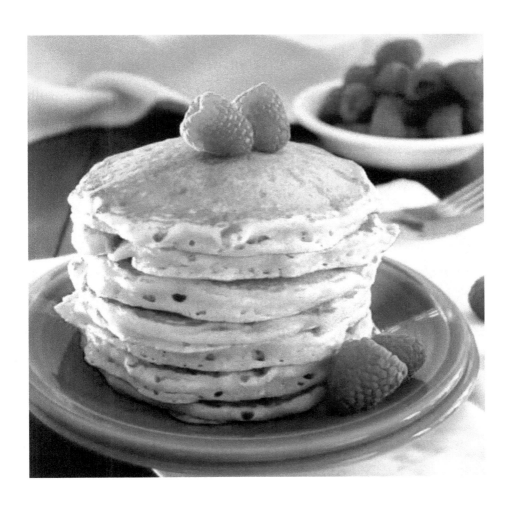

Upside Down 3-Level Apple Nut Cake

Preparation time: 15 minutes Cooking time: 45 minutes 6 Servings.

Ingredients:

2 sliced apples 2 ½ cups all-purpose flour 1 tsp. salt 1 tsp. baking powder 1 ½ cup diced pecans 1 tsp. vanilla 1 ½ tsp. cinnamon ½ cup vegan butter 1/3 cup maple syrup ½ cup applesauce

Directions:

Begin by preheating your oven to 350 degrees Fahrenheit. Next, prepare an 8x8 cake pan. Pour one tbsp.. of the maple syrup over the bottom of the pan. Next, add a layer of apples at the bottom followed by a layer of pecans. Utilize half of both. Next, mix together all the dry ingredients in a separate bowl. Add the wet ingredients to the dry ingredients, and stir well. Add half of this created batter to the cake pan. Next, add another layer of apples followed by another layer of pecans. Spread the remaining batter over the pecans, and allow the cake to bake for fifty-five minutes. Allow the cake to coo for twenty minutes, and enjoy!

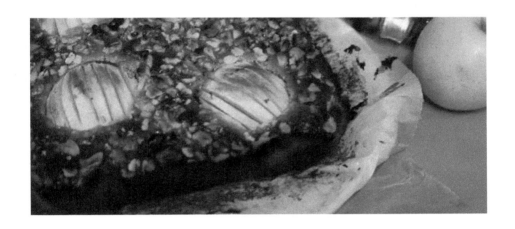

Banana Cinnamon Smoothie

Cooking time: 0 minutes Preparation time: 30 minutes Servings: 01

Ingredients:

1 cup unsweetened almond milk ½ cup oats 1 banana 1 tablespoon peanut butter ½ teaspoon cinnamon A drizzle of maple syrup

Directions:

Add all the ingredients to a blender. Hit the pulse button and blend till it is smooth. Chill well to serve.

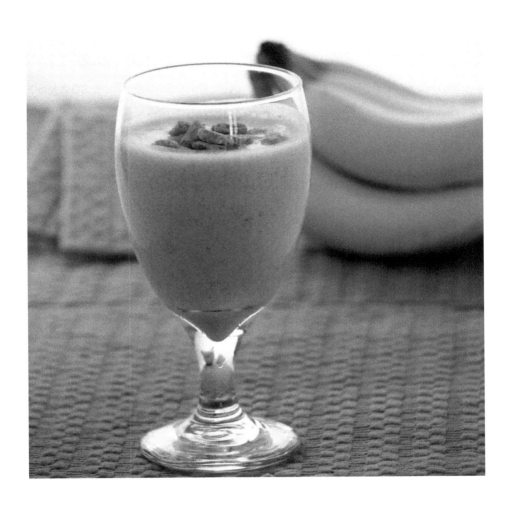

Green Glass Smoothie

Preparation time: 30 minutes Cooking time: 0 minutes Servings: 01

Ingredients:

1 cup baby spinach ½ cup cucumber, chopped 1 celery stalk ½ medium banana ½ cup pineapple 6 oz soy yogurt ¼ cup flax ½ cup of water 4 ice cubes

Directions:

Add all the ingredients to a blender. Hit the pulse button and blend till it is smooth. Chill well to serve.

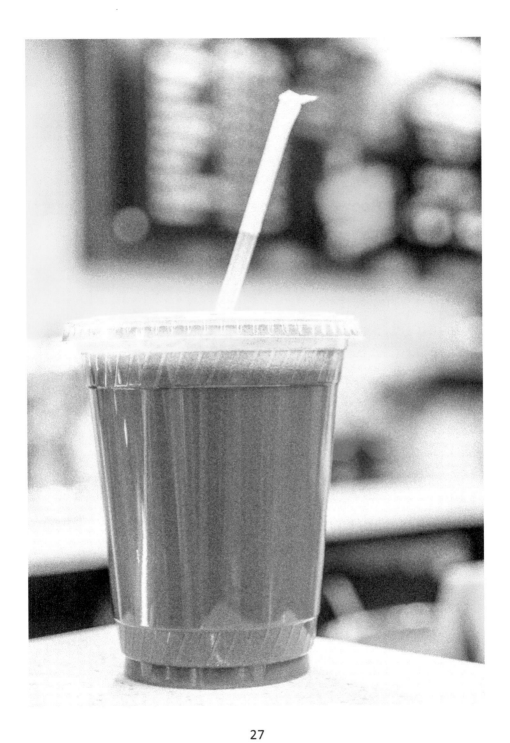

Beet Cinnamon Smoothie

Preparation time: 30 minutes Cooking time: 0 minutes Servings: 01

Ingredients:

2 cups almond milk ½ of a beet, cooked 3 tablespoons raw cacao powder 3-6 dates, pitted ½ teaspoon vanilla extract ¼ teaspoon ground cinnamon 1 pinch of salt

Directions:

Add all ingredients to a blender. Hit the pulse button and blend till it is smooth.

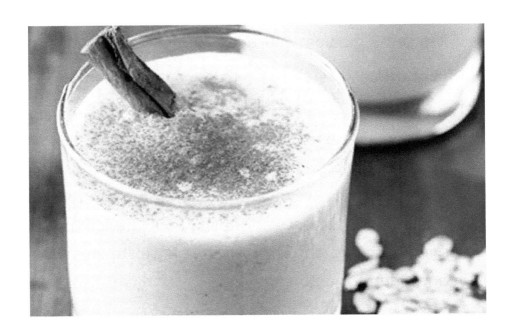

Avocado chocolate mousse

Preparation time: 5 minutes | Cooking time: 5 minutes | Servings: 4

Ingredients:

½ cup maple syrup 2/3 cup cocoa powder ¼ cup coconut cream 1tsp vanilla extract ½ cup vegan chocolate chips ¼ tsp salt 2 medium avocado

Directions:

Take a blender, pour maple syrup, coconut cream, cocoa powder, vanilla extract and blend well. Melt the chocolate chip into the microwave and pour into blender. Blend the mixture for a few seconds. In the end, add avocado and blend until turn smooth and thick. Pour the mixture into serving cups and garnish with the chocolate chips. Keep in a refrigerator before serving.

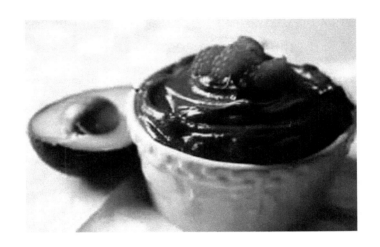

Gluten-free lemon cake

Preparation time: 25 minutes | Cooking time: 42 minutes | Servings: 16 slices

Ingredients:

For cake: 1 cup of vegetable oil 4 large eggs 1 ½ cup granulated sugar 2 ½ cup gluten-free flour ½ tsp salt 3 tsp baking powder gluten-free 1 cup milk 2 tsp lemon extract 1 medium lemon zest

For frosting: 1 cup butter 6 cups powdered sugar ¼ cup lemon juice ½ cup lemon curd

Directions:

For cake:

Preheat the oven first at 350 degrees. Prepare the baking pan with flour dust and set aside. Take a bowl, add sugar and oil to mix. Now beat the eggs in a better for a minute, then add flour, salt, baking powder, milk, lemon extract and lemon zest. Beat all the Ingredients for a minute. Mix them with sugar and oil. Now take the baking pan, spread the batter evenly into the pan. Bake it for around 28 to 32 minutes. Take out the cake from the oven, separate its sides from the pan and set it in a cooking rack. For frosting: Take a medium bowl, pour butter and mix well until smooth. Gradually add the powdered sugar and mix.

Add the 1tbsp lemon juice and mix it well. Beat until the desired consistency obtained. Now cut the cake from the center and spread the frosting inside evenly. Now put the other portion on top and covered sides and top with the frosting and evenly spread out with a spatula. Garnish with the lemon curd on the top and chill before serving.

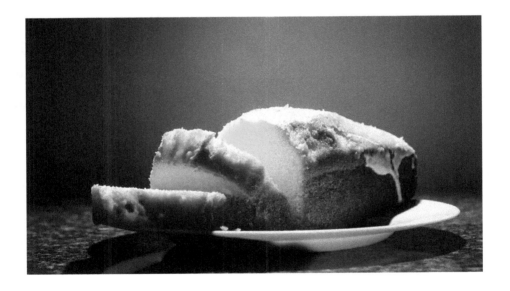

No-bake pumpkin pie

Preparation time: 10 minutes | Cooking time: 1 hour | Servings: 8

Ingredients:

1 cup pumpkin puree 2 tsp pumpkin pie spice 3.4 oz. vanilla pudding 8-ounce cool whip ¼ cup milk 1 graham cracker crust Whipped cream for garnish

Directions:

Take a bowl pour pumpkin puree in it, add pudding mix, pumpkin pie spice and milk. Mix the Ingredients well until they turn smooth. Now fold it into cool whip carefully. Take a graham cracker in a pie pan and spread the pumpkin puree on the pie and spread well. Chill it well before serving, and serve with whipped cream topping.

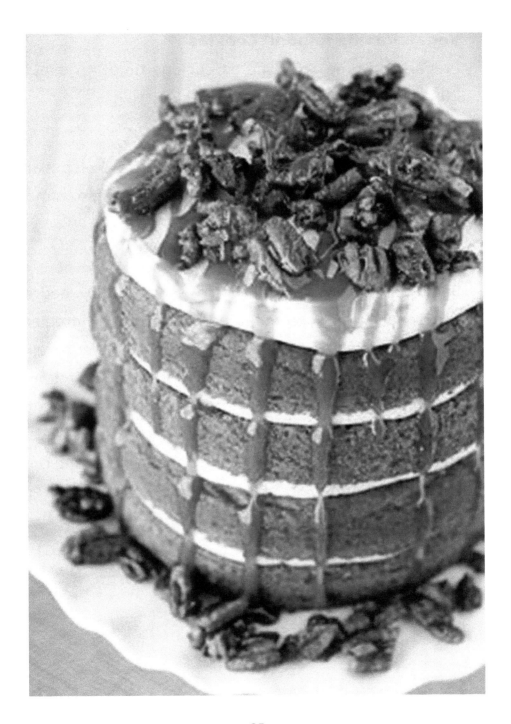

Vegan Vanilla Almond Cookies

Preparation time: 15 minutes Cooking time: 45 minutes 20 cookies.

Ingredients:

2 cups all-purpose flour 1 cup almond meal ½ tsp. salt 1 cup powdered sugar 1 cup vegan butter ½ tsp. almond extract 2 tsp. vanilla 20 almonds

Directions:

Begin by preheating your oven to 350 degrees Fahrenheit. Next, you mix together your dry ingredients in a large bowl. Add the wet ingredients, and stir well to create a dough. Don't add the almonds. Next, roll your dough into a log with a two-inch diameter, and slice the cookie roll into flat cookies—like you would slice a cucumber. Place the cookies on a baking sheet, and press the almonds into the cookies. Bake the cookies for twenty minutes in the preheated oven, and enjoy.

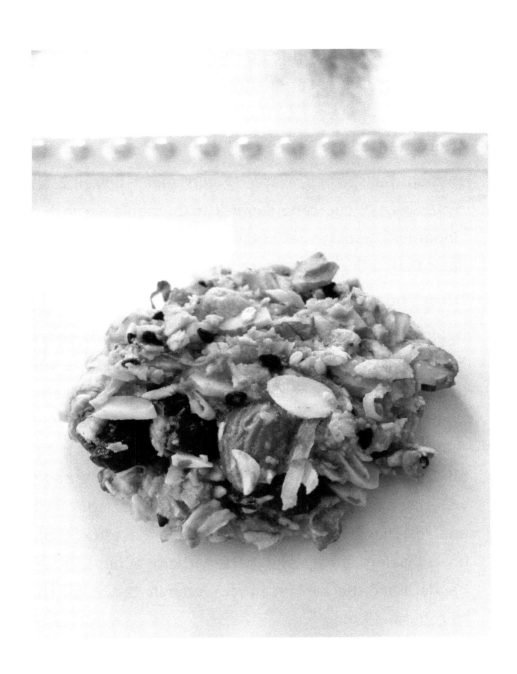

Vegan Lover's Ginger Cookies

Preparation time: 15 minutes Cooking time: 55 minutes 12 Cookies.

Ingredients:

½ tbsp. flax 2 tbsp. water ¼ cup vegan butter 2 tbsp. molasses 1/3 cup cane sugar 2 tbsp. maple syrup 1 tsp. cinnamon 1 tsp. ginger ½ tsp. baking soda 1 ½ cups light spelt flour 1/3 cup diced candied ginger 2 tbsp. sugar

Directions:

Begin by preheating your oven to 350 degrees Fahrenheit. Next, bring together the flax and the water in a small bowl. Set it aside and allow it to thicken for five minutes. Next, beat together the vegan butter, the molasses, the sugar, the vanilla, the syrup, and the flax mixture. Add the dry ingredients to this mixture and stir well. Lastly, add the candied ginger. Create cookie balls and roll them in the 2 tbsp. of sugar. Place the cookies on a baking sheet, and flatten them a bit with your hands. Bake the cookies for twelve minutes. Allow them to cool, and enjoy!

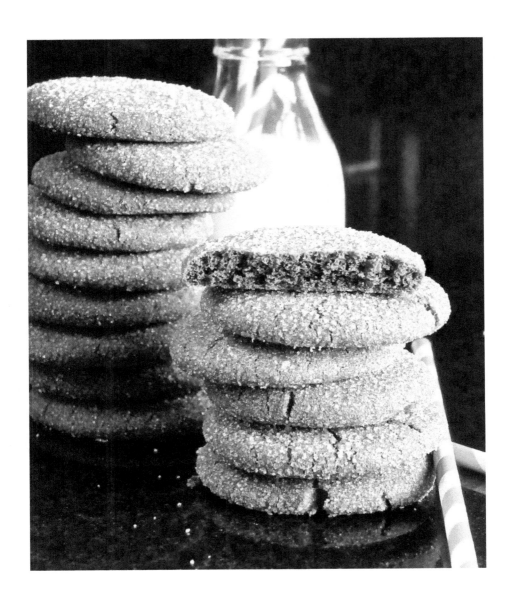

Elementary Party Vegan Oatmeal Raisin Cookies

Preparation time: 15 minutes Cooking time: 35 minutes 24 cookies.

Ingredients:

1 cup whole wheat flour ½ tsp. salt ½ tsp. baking soda 1 tsp. cinnamon ½ cup brown sugar 2 tbsp. maple syrup ½ cup sugar 1/3 cup applesauce ½ tsp. vanilla 1/3 cup olive oil ½ cup raisins 1 ¾ cup oats

Directions: Begin by preheating the oven to 350 degrees Fahrenheit. Next, mix together all the dry ingredients. Place this mixture to the side. Next, mix together all the wet ingredients in a large mixing bowl. Add the dry ingredients to the wet ingredients slowly, stirring as you go. Add the oats next, stirring well. Lastly, add the raisins. Allow the batter to chill in the refrigerator for twenty minutes. Afterwards, drop the cookies onto a baking sheet and bake them for thirteen minutes. Enjoy after cooling. Classic

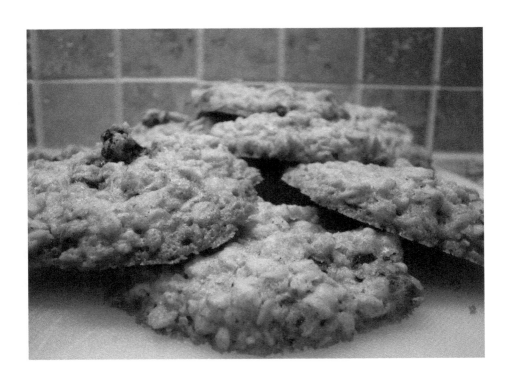

Granola Grammar Muffins

Preparation time: 15 minutes Cooking time: 35 minutes 16 muffins.

Ingredients:

1 cup granola ¼ cup oat flour 1 cup all-purpose flour 1 cup whole wheat flour 1 cup diced walnuts 2 tbsp. flax seed 6 bsp. Water ½ cup chocolate chips 1 tsp. baking soda 2 tsp. baking powder 2 cups applesauce ½ cup soymilk ½ cup brown sugar 2 tbsp. melted coconut oil

Directions:

Begin by preheating your oven to 400 degrees Fahrenheit. Next, bring together the flax seed and the water and set them to the side in order to thicken. Next, mix together all the dry ingredients. Mix the wet ingredients separately, adding the flax seed and water mixture after it has thickened. Next, bring the two mixtures together and stir well. Pour the batter into muffin tins, and bake the muffins for twenty minutes. Allow the muffins to cool, and enjoy.

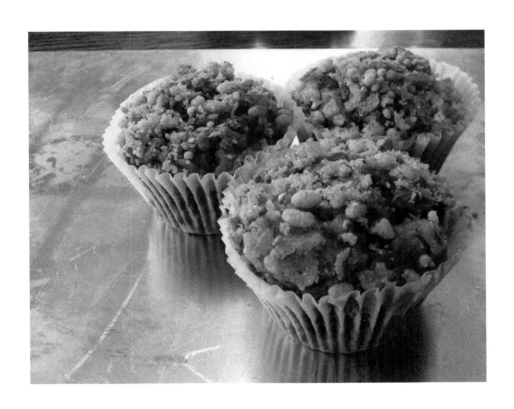

Careful Carrot Muffin

Preparation time: 15 minutes Cooking time: 35 minutes 20 muffins.

Ingredients:

1 ¼ cup whole-wheat flour 2 cups bran flakes ½ cup coconut palm sugar 1 tsp. baking soda 1 tsp. cinnamon 1 tsp. baking powder 1 cup grated carrots 1 zest of an orange ½ tsp. salt ½ cup diced walnuts 1/3 cup raisins 2 cups almond milk 2 tsp. vinegar 1/3 cup avocado oil 1 tsp. apple cider vinegar

Directions:

Begin by preheating your oven to 400 degrees Fahrenheit. Next, mix together all the dry ingredients in a large bowl. Mix the wet ingredients together in a smaller bowl, and then add the wet ingredients to the dry ingredients, stirring slowly. Next, fill the muffin tins with your batter, and bake the muffins for twenty minutes. Cool the muffins, and enjoy!

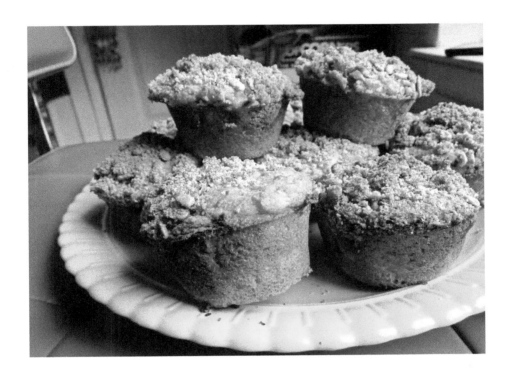

Pull-Apart Vegan Monkey Bread

Preparation time: 15 minutes Cooking time: 45 minutes 16 pieces.

Ingredients:

First part: 2 cups whole-wheat flour 1 tbsp. baking powder 1/3 cup sugar 1 tsp. salt 6 tbsp. vegan butter Second part: 1 cup nondairy chocolate chips 1 cup soymilk Third part: 1/3 cup sugar 2 tsp. cinnamon 3 tbsp. melted vegan butter

Directions:

Begin by preheating your oven to 350 degrees Fahrenheit. Next, mix together the first part's ingredients. Cut the butter into the dry ingredients. Next, mix all the second part's ingredients together into the first mixture. This should create a dough. Next, create sixteen dough balls to splay in the bread pan. The dough balls should touch each other. Then drizzle the balls with melted butter. Mix together the sugar and the cinnamon, and sprinkle this creation over the monkey bread. Bake the monkey bread for thirty minutes. Allow the bread to cool for a few minutes, and then eat up immediately. Enjoy!

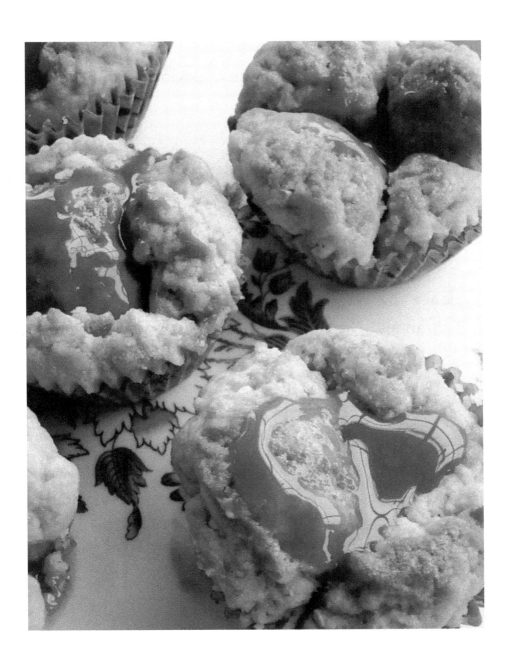

Banana Blueberry Bread

Preparation time: 15 minutes Cooking time: 35 minutes 8 Servings.

Ingredients:

3 tbsp. lemon juice 4 bananas ½ cup agave nectar ½ cup vegan milk 1 ¾ cup all-purpose flour 1 tsp. baking soda 1 tsp. baking powder 1 tsp. salt 2 cups blueberries

Directions:

Begin by preheating your oven to 350 degrees Fahrenheit. Next, mix together the dry ingredients in a large bowl and your wet ingredients in a different, smaller bowl. Make sure to mash up the bananas well. Stir the ingredients together in the large bowl, making sure to completely assimilate the ingredients together. Add the blueberries last, and then pour the mixture into a bread pan. Allow the bread to bake for fifty minutes, and enjoy.

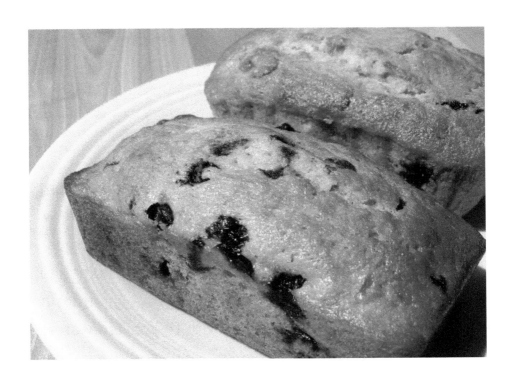

Vegan Lemon Meringue Pie

Preparation time: 15 minutes Cooking time: 45 minutes 8 slices.

Ingredients:

1 ½ cups sugar 1/3 up cornstarch ½ tsp. salt ½ tsp. agar 1 cup water 1 ½ cup coconut milk 2 tbsp. lemon zest 1 cup lemon juice Meringue Ingredients: 10 tbsp. egg replacer 5 tbsp. chilled water 1 ¼ cup sugar 1 prepared pie crust (store bought) Lemon Pie

Directions:

Begin by adding the first group of ingredients: from the sugar to the lemon juice, to the saucepan. Allow the mixture to boil, stirring all the time. After it becomes very thick, pour the mixture into the pie pan. Next, preheat the oven to 210 degrees Fahrenheit. In a separate bowl, mix together the egg replacer with the chilled water. Stir well, creating soft white peaks. Now, add the sugar. Mix slowly so that the meringue is super-thick and will refuse to fall down if tipped over. Next, scoop this meringue over the chilled lemon filling, prepared above, and then allow the pie to sit for twenty minutes. Now, allow the pie to cook in the oven for thirty minutes. Allow the pie to cool after baking, and serve. Enjoy.

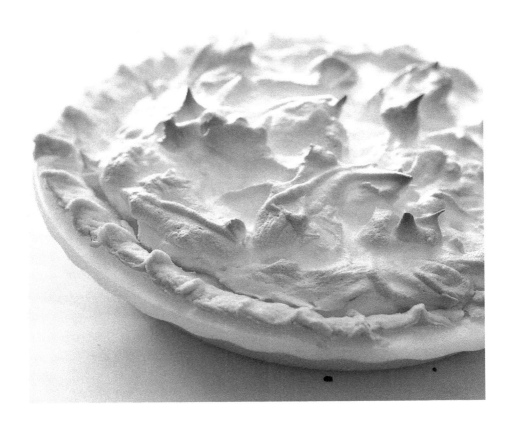

Vegan Vanilla Ice Cream

Preparation time: 15 minutes Cooking time: 45 minutes 2 cups.

Ingredients:

3 vanilla pods 1 ½ tsp. vanilla bean paste 400 ml soymilk 600 grams light coconut milk 200 grams agave syrup

Directions: Begin by slicing the vanilla pods and removing the seeds. Place the seeds in a big mixing bowl and toss out the pods. Next, add the rest of the ingredients, and position the ingredients into an ice cream maker. Churn the ice cream for forty-five minutes. Next, place the mixture into a freezer container, and allow the ice cream to freeze for three hours. Serve, and enjoy!

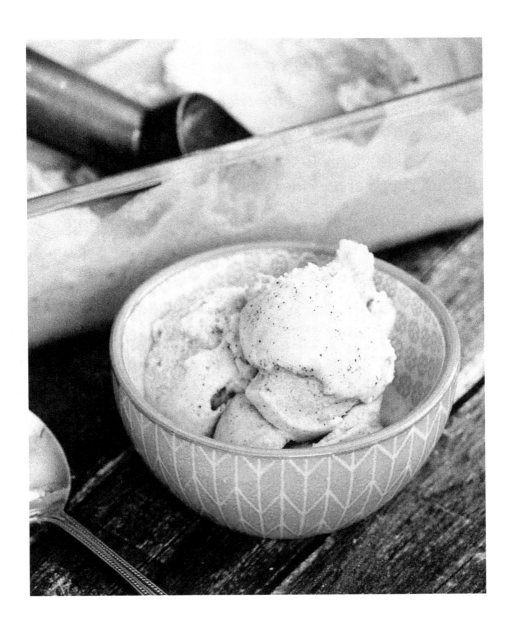

Vegan Cupcakes

Preparation time: 15 minutes Cooking time: 55 minutes Servings: 5

Ingredients:

1 ¼ tsp vanilla extract ½ tsp salt 2 tsp baking soda 5 tbsp. Splenda 1 ½ cups almond milk ½ cup coconut oil, warmed until liquid ½ tsp baking powder 2 cups almond flour 1 tbsp apple cider vinegar

Directions: Set the oven at 350 degrees. Spread oil or butter on 12 muffin tins. You can also cover it with paper liners if desired. Pour the apple cider in a cup. Add enough almond milk to make it 1 ½ cups. Set it aside for 5 minutes until it curdles. Whisk the flour, baking powder, salt, sugar and baking soda. Pour the mixture to the dry mixture and whisk to combine. Scoop the batter into the muffin tins. Bake for 15-20 minutes until it is done. Remove from the oven and let it cool in a wire rack. Arrange in a platter and decorate it as desired.

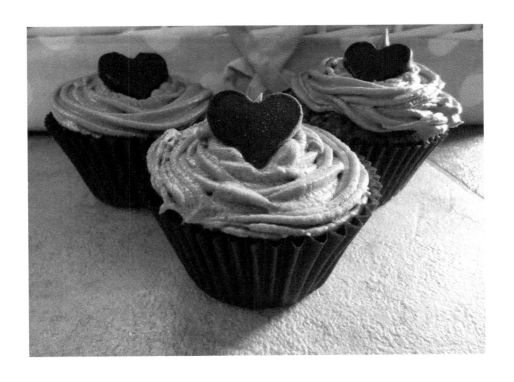

Lemon Bars

Preparation time: 15 minutes Cooking time: 25 minutes
Servings: 5

Ingredients:

3/4 cup melted butter 3/4 cup almond flour 1 1/2 cups
boiling water 2/3 cup lemon gelatin mix, no sugar added
3 Tbsp freshly squeezed lemon juice 12 oz cream cheese

Directions:

Set the oven to 350 degrees F. Combine the melted
butter and flour together in a bowl, then pour the mixture
into a baking pan, pressing down to create a crust. Bake
for 10 minutes then set on a cooling rack. Cool
completely before use. In a large mixing bowl, mix the
gelatin and boiling water. Stir until the gelatin completely
dissolves. Stir in the lemon juice and cream cheese,
mixing well. Pour the mixture on top of the crust, then
place in the refrigerator and chill overnight, or for 3 hours
at least. Slice into 12 servings.

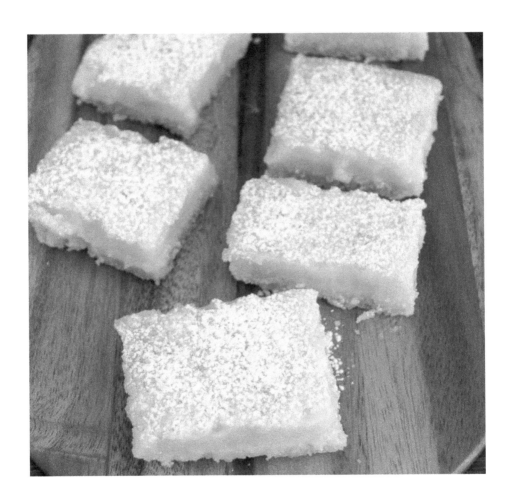

Chocolate Peanut Butter Smoothie

Preparation time: 30 minutes Cooking time: 0 minutes Servings: 01

Ingredients:

1 cup almond milk ¼ cup quick oats 1 scoop plant-based protein powder 2 tablespoons peanut butter 2 teaspoons cocoa powder 1 tablespoon maple syrup 1 cup ice

Directions: Add all ingredients to a blender. Hit the pulse button and blend till it is smooth. Chill well to serve.

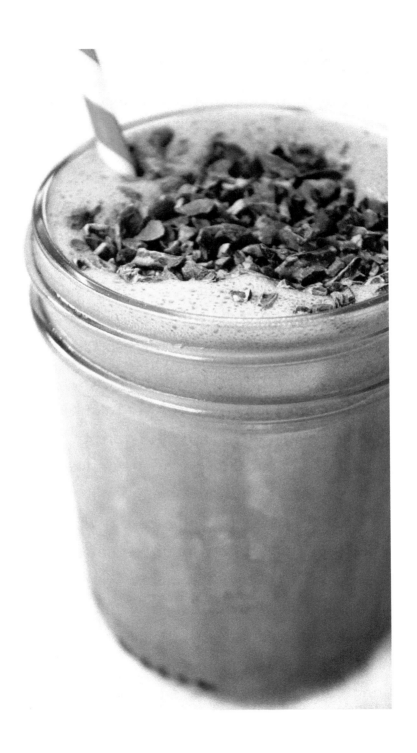

Carrot cake muffins

Preparation time: 10 minutes | Cooking time: 20 minutes | Servings: 12 muffins

Ingredients:

For muffins:

1 cup brown sugar 2 eggs ½ cup of vegetable oil 1 cup carrots shredded ½ cup milk 1 ½ cup flour 1 tsp baking powder 1 tsp baking soda 1 tsp cinnamon ¼ tsp salt Frosting: ¼ cup butter ¼ cup cream cheese 2 ½ cup icing sugar ¼ tsp vanilla Salt a pinch 2tbsp Cream

Directions: Preheat oven at 400 degrees. Set the muffin pan with oil grease and flour dust. Take a medium bowl and whisk vegetable oil, eggs, carrot, and milk. In another bowl, mix the dry Ingredients like sugar, flour, baking powder, baking soda, cinnamon and salt. Now mix the dry Ingredients into the batter with the help of spatula until smooth. Now pour the batter into a muffin pan and bake it for 20 minutes. Prepare the cream frosting in a bowl by adding the butter, icing sugar, cream cheese, cream, salt and vanilla extract, beat them until frothy. Serve the muffin with the cream cheese frosting.

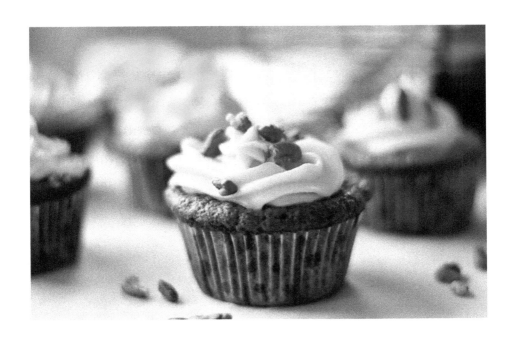

Peanut butter stuffed dates

Preparation time: 5 minutes | Cooking time: 5 minutes | Servings: 6

Ingredients:

6 medjool dates 6tsp peanut butter Chocolate crunches or coconut for topping

Directions:

Take 6 dates, wash them and let them dry. Now remove the pits from the dates without splitting them into half. Fill each date with a tablespoon of peanut butter. Set them in the refrigerator to get cold for a while. Now cut the dates from the center half. Top each with different topping and serve chilled.

and refrigerate for 5 hours. Cut it into sixteen bars and serve.

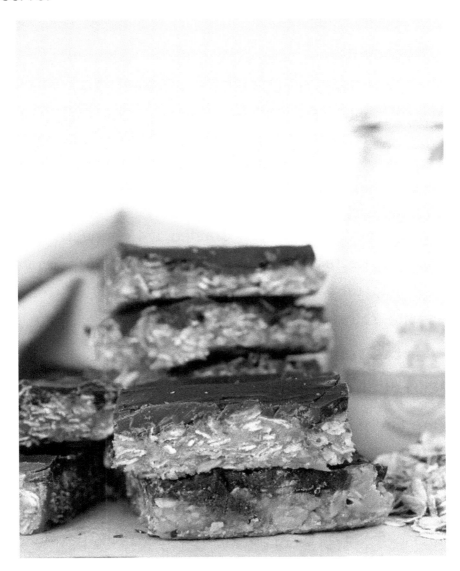

Lemon Cashew Tart

Preparation time:3 hours and15 minutes Cooking time:0 minuteServings: 12

Ingredients:

For the Crust: 1 cup almonds 4 dates, pitted, soaked in warm water for 10 minutes in water, drained 1/8 teaspoon crystal salt 1 teaspoon vanilla extract, unsweetened

For the Cream: 1 cup cashews, soaked in warm water for 10 minutes in water, drained 1/4 cup water 1/4 cup coconut nectar 1 teaspoon coconut oil 1 teaspoon vanilla extract, unsweetened 1 lemon, Juiced 1/8 teaspoon crystal salt

For the Topping: Shredded coconut as needed

Directions:

Prepare the cream and for this, place all its ingredients in a food processor, pulse for 2 minutes until smooth, and then refrigerate for 1 hour. Then prepare the crust, and for this, place all its ingredients in a food processor and pulse for 3 to 5 minutes until the thick paste comes together. Take a tart pan, grease it with oil, place crust mixture in it and spread and press the mixture evenly in the bottom and along the sides, and freeze until required.

Pour the filling into the prepared tart, smooth the top, and refrigerate for 2 hours until set. Cut tart into slices and then serve.

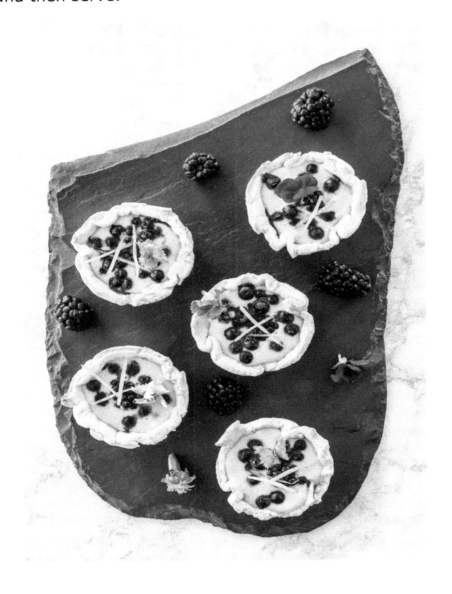

Caramel Brownie Slice

Preparation time: 4 hours Cooking time: 0 minute Servings: 16

Ingredients:

For the Base: ¼ cup dried figs 1 cup dried dates ½ cup cacao powder ½ cup pecans ½ cup walnuts

For the Caramel Layer: ¼ teaspoons sea salt 2 cups dried dates, soaked in water for 1 hour 3 Tablespoons coconut oil 5 Tablespoons water

For the Chocolate Topping: 1/3 cup agave nectar ½ cup cacao powder ¼ cup of coconut oil

Directions:

Prepare the base, and for this, place all its ingredients in a food processor and pulse for 3 to 5 minutes until the thick paste comes together. Take an 8 by 8 inches baking dish, grease it with oil, place base mixture in it and spread and press the mixture evenly in the bottom, and freeze until required. Prepare the caramel layer, and for this, place all its ingredients in a food processor and pulse for 2 minutes until smooth. Pour the caramel into the prepared baking dish, smooth the top and freeze for 20 minutes. Then prepare the topping and for this, place all its ingredients in a food processor, and pulse for 1 minute until combined. Gently spread the chocolate mixture over the caramel layer and then freeze for 3 hours until set. Serve straight away.

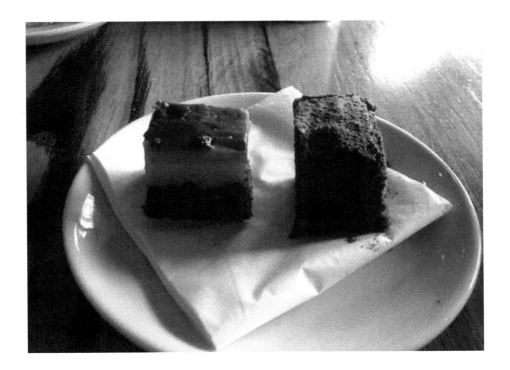

Double Chocolate Orange Cheesecake

Preparation time: 4 hours Cooking time: 0 minute Servings: 12

Ingredients:

For the Base: 9 Medjool dates, pitted 1/3 cup Brazil nuts 2 tablespoons maple syrup 1/3 cup walnuts 2 tablespoons water 3 tablespoons cacao powder

For the Chocolate Cheesecake: 1/2 cup cacao powder 1 1/2 cups cashews, soaked for 10 minutes in warm water, drained 1/3 cup liquid coconut oil 1 teaspoon vanilla extract, unsweetened 1/3 cup maple syrup 1/3 cup water

For the Orange Cheesecake:

2 oranges, juiced 1/4 cup maple syrup 1 cup cashews, soaked for 10 minutes in warm water, drained 1 teaspoon vanillaextract, unsweetened 2 tablespoons coconut butter 1/2 cup liquid coconut oil 2 oranges, zested 4 drops of orange essential oil

For the Chocolate Topping: 3 tablespoons cacao powder 3 drops of orange essential oil 2 tablespoons liquid coconut oil 3 tablespoons maple syrup

Directions:

Prepare the base, and for this, place all its ingredients in a food processor and pulse for 3 to 5 minutes until the thick paste comes together. Take a cake tin, place crust mixture in it and spread and press the mixture evenly in the bottom, and freeze until required. Prepare the chocolate cheesecake, and for this, place all its ingredients in a food processor and pulse for 2 minutes until smooth. Pour the chocolate cheesecake mixture on top of the prepared base, smooth the top and freeze for 20 minutes until set. Then prepare the orange cheesecake and for this, place all its ingredients in a food processor, and pulse for 2 minutes until smooth Top orange cheesecake mixture over chocolate cheesecake, and then freeze for 3 hours until hardened. Then prepare the chocolate topping and for this, take a bowl, add all the ingredients in it and stir until well combined. Spread chocolate topping over the top, freeze the cake for 10 minutes until the topping has hardened and then slice to serve.

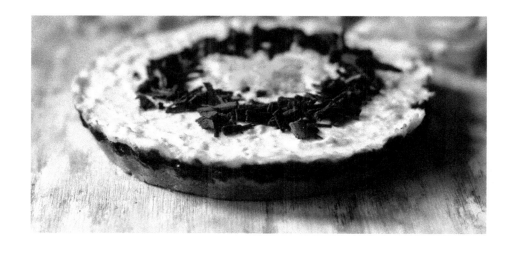

Matcha Coconut Cream Pie

Preparation time: 5 minutes Cooking time: 0 minute Servings: 4

Ingredients:

For the Crust: 1/2 cup ground flaxseed 3/4 cup shredded dried coconut 1 cup Medjool dates, pitted 3/4 cup dehydrated buckwheat groats 1/4 teaspoons sea salt

For the Filling: 1 cup dried coconut flakes 4 cups of coconut meat 1/4 cup and 2 Tablespoons coconut nectar 1/2 Tablespoons vanilla extract, unsweetened 1/4 teaspoons sea salt 2/3 cup and 2 Tablespoons coconut butter 1 Tablespoons matcha powder 1/2 cup coconut water

Directions:

Prepare the crust, and for this, place all its ingredients in a food processor and pulse for 3 to 5 minutes until the thick paste comes together. Take a 6-inch springform pan, grease it with oil, place crust mixture in it and spread and press the mixture evenly in the bottom and along the sides, and freeze until required. Prepare the filling and for this, place all its ingredients in a food processor, and pulse for 2 minutes until smooth. Pour the filling into prepared pan, smooth the top, and freeze for 4 hours until set. Cut pie into slices and then serve.

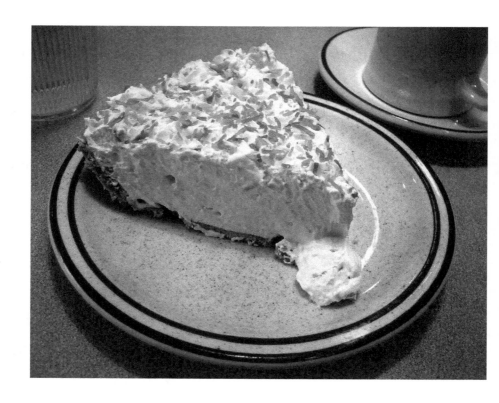

Chocolate Raspberry Brownies

Preparation time: 4 hours Cooking time: 0 minute Servings: 4

Ingredients:

For the Chocolate Brownie Base: 12 Medjool Dates, pitted 3/4 cup oat flour 3/4 cup almond meal 3 tablespoons cacao 1 teaspoon vanilla extract, unsweetened 1/8 teaspoon sea salt 3 tablespoons water 1/2 cup pecans, chopped

For the Raspberry Cheesecake: 3/4 cup cashews, soaked, drained 6 tablespoons agave nectar 1/2 cup raspberries 1 teaspoon vanilla extract, unsweetened 1 lemon, juiced 6 tablespoons liquid coconut oil

For the Chocolate Coating: 2 1/2 tablespoons cacao powder 3 3/4 tablespoons coconut Oil 2 tablespoons maple syrup 1/8 teaspoon sea salt

Directions:

Prepare the crust, and for this, place all its ingredients in a food processor and pulse for 3 to 5 minutes until the thick paste comes together. Take a 6-inch springform pan, grease it with oil, place crust mixture in it and spread and press the mixture evenly in the bottom and along the sides, and freeze until required. Prepare the cheesecake topping, and for this, place all its ingredients in a food processor and pulse for 2 minutes until smooth. Pour the filling into prepared pan, smooth the top, and freeze for 8 hours until solid. Prepare the chocolate coating and for this, whisk together all its ingredients until smooth, drizzle on top of the cake and then serve.

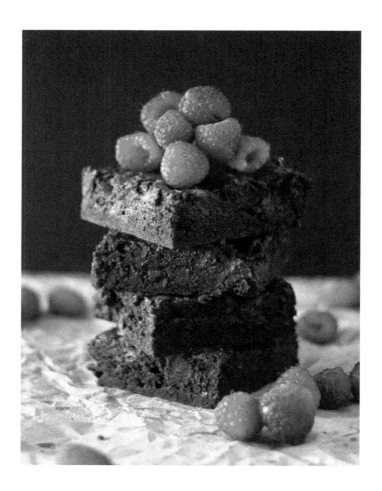

Strawberry Mousse

Preparation time: 5 minutes Cooking time: 15 minutes Servings: 4

Ingredients:

8 ounces coconut milk, unsweetened 2 tablespoons honey 5 strawberries

Directions:

Place berries in a blender and pulse until the smooth mixture comes together. Place milk in a bowl, whisk until whipped, and then add remaining ingredients and stir until combined. Refrigerate the mousse for 10 minutes and then serve.

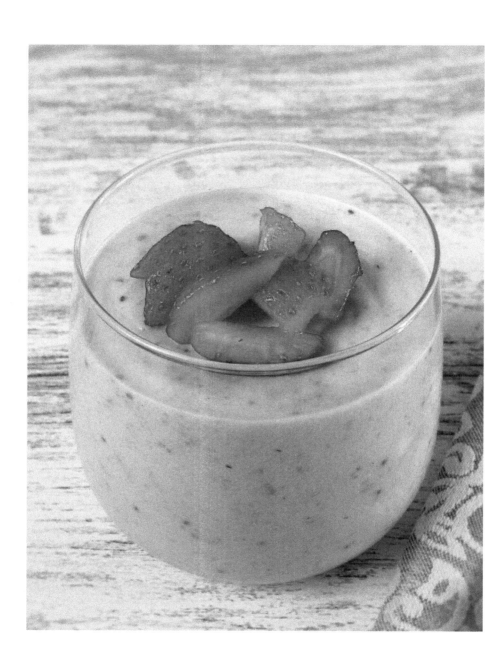

Green Goddess Hummus

Preparation time: 5 minutes Cooking time: 0 minute Servings: 6

Ingredients:

¼ cup tahini ¼ cup lemon juice 2 tablespoons olive oil ½ cup chopped parsley ¼ cup chopped basil 3 tablespoons chopped chives 1 large clove of garlic, peeled, chopped ½ teaspoon salt 15-ounce cooked chickpeas 2 tablespoons water

Directions:

Place all the ingredients in the order in a food processor or blender and then pulse for 3 to 5 minutes at high speed until the thick mixture comes together. Tip the hummus in a bowl and then serve.

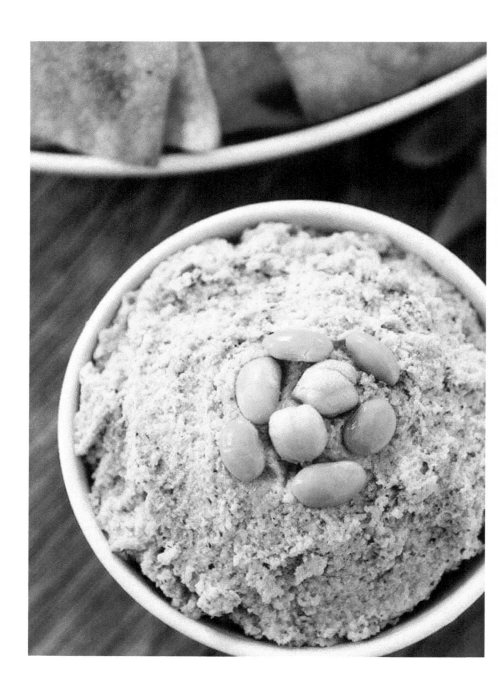

Tomato Jam

Preparation time: 10 minutes Cooking time: 20 minutes
Servings: 16

Ingredients:

2 pounds tomatoes ¼ teaspoon. ground black pepper ½
teaspoon. salt ¼ cup coconut sugar ½ teaspoon. white
wine vinegar ¼ teaspoon. smoked paprika

Directions:

Place a large pot filled with water over medium heat,
bring it to boil, then add tomatoes and boil for 1 minute.
Transfer tomatoes to a bowl containing chilled water, let
them stand for 2 minutes, and then peel them by hand.
Cut the tomatoes, remove and discard seeds, then chop
tomatoes and place them in a large pot. Sprinkle sugar
over coconut, stir until mixed and let it stand for 10
minutes. Then place the pot over medium-high heat,
cook for 15 minutes, then add remaining ingredients
except for vinegar and cook for 10 minutes until
thickened. Remove pot from heat, stir in vinegar and
serve.

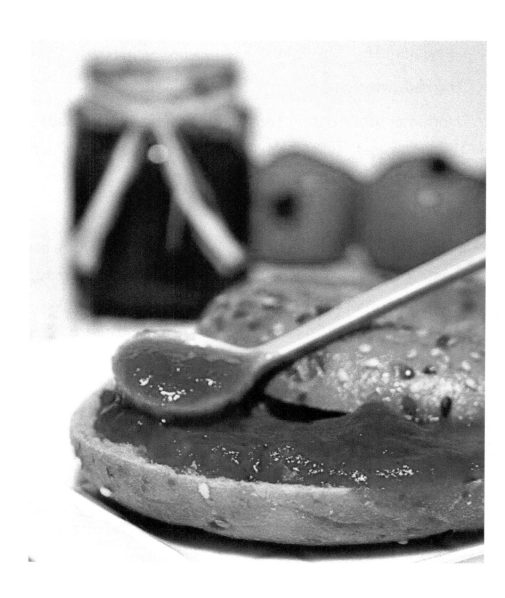

Buffalo Chicken Dip

Preparation time: 5 minutes Cooking time: 15 minutes Servings: 4

Ingredients:

2 cups cashews 2 teaspoons garlic powder 1 1/2 teaspoons salt 2 teaspoons onion powder 3 tablespoons lemon juice 1 cup buffalo sauce 1 cup of water 14-ounce artichoke hearts, packed in water, drained

Directions:

Switch on the oven, then set it to 375 degrees F and let it preheat. Meanwhile, pour 3 cups of boiling water in a bowl, add cashews and let soak for 5 minutes. Then drain the cashew, transfer them into the blender, pour in water, add lemon juice and all the seasoning and blend until smooth. Add artichokes and buffalo sauce, process until chunky mixture comes together, and then transfer the dip to an ovenproof dish. Bake for 20 minutes and then serve.

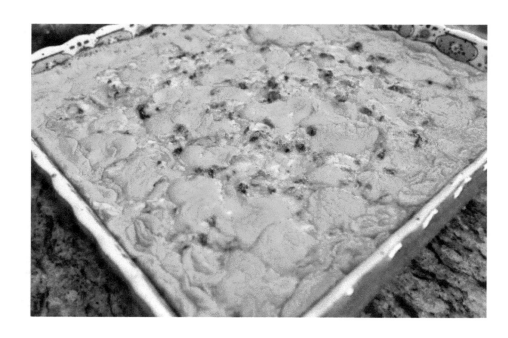

Vegan Ranch Dressing

Preparation time: 5 minutes Cooking time: 0 minute Servings: 16

Ingredients:

1/4 teaspoon. ground black pepper 2 teaspoon. chopped parsley 1/2 teaspoon. garlic powder 1 tablespoon chopped dill 1/2 teaspoon. onion powder 1 cup vegan mayonnaise 1/2 cup soy milk, unsweetened

Directions:

Take a medium bowl, add all the ingredients in it and then whisk until combined. Serve straight away

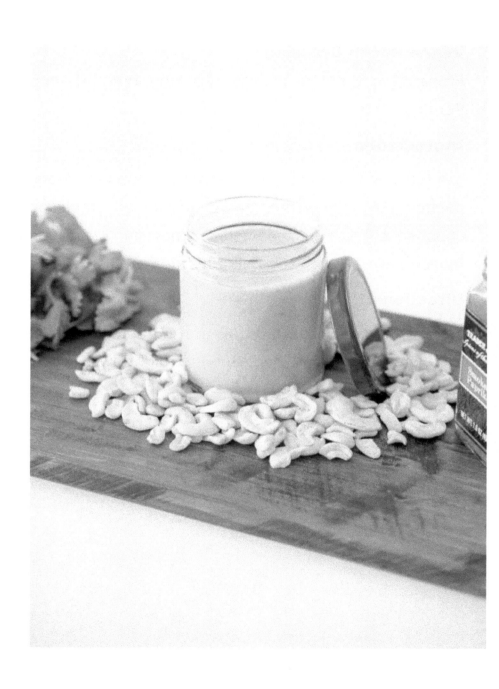

Nacho Cheese Sauce

Preparation time: 15 minutes Cooking time: 5 minutes
Servings: 12

Ingredients:

2 cups cashews, unsalted , soaked in warm water for 15 minutes 2 teaspoons salt 1/2 cup nutritional yeast 1 teaspoon garlic powder 1/2 teaspoon smoked paprika 1/2 teaspoon red chili powder 1 teaspoon onion powder 2 teaspoons Sriracha 3 tablespoons lemon juice 4 cups water, divided

Directions:

Drain the cashews, transfer them to a food processor, then add remaining ingredients, reserving 3 cups water, and , and pulse for 3 minutes until smooth. Tip the mixture in a saucepan, place it over medium heat and cook for 3 to 5 minutes until the sauce has thickened and bubbling, whisking constantly. When done, taste the sauce to adjust seasoning and then serve.

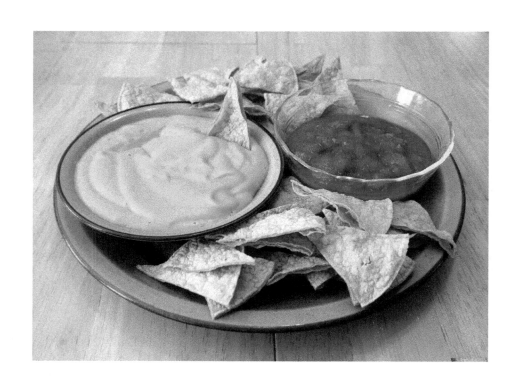

Garlic Alfredo Sauce

Preparation time: 10 minutes Cooking time: 5 minutes
Servings: 4

Ingredients:

1 1/2 cups cashews, unsalted , soaked in warm water for 15 minutes 6 cloves of garlic, peeled, minced 1/2 medium sweet onion, peeled, chopped 1 teaspoon salt 1/4 cup nutritional yeast 1 tablespoon lemon juice 2 tablespoons olive oil 2 cups almond milk, unsweetened 12 ounces fettuccine pasta, cooked, for serving

Directions:

Take a small saucepan, place it over medium heat, add oil and when hot, add onion and garlic, and cook for 5 minutes until sauté. Meanwhile, drain the cashews, transfer them into a food processor, add remaining ingredients including onion mixture, except for pasta, and pulse for 3 minutes until very smooth. Pour the prepared sauce over pasta, toss until coated and serve.

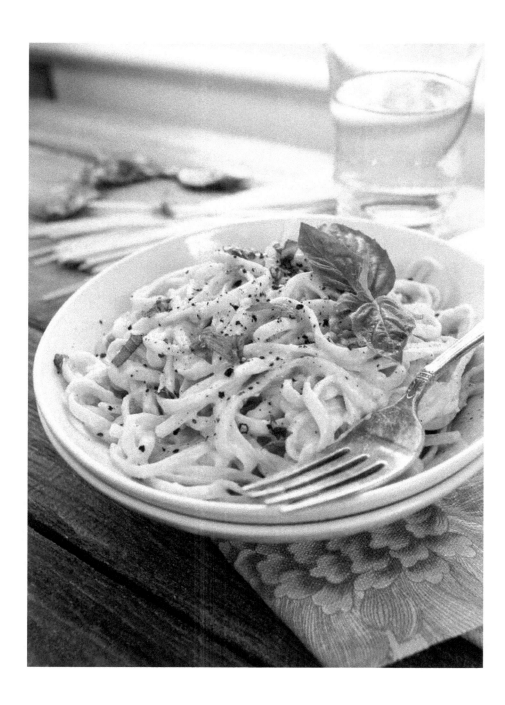

Garden Greens & Yogurt Shake

Preparation time: 5 minutes Cooking time: 0 minutes Servings: 1

Ingredients:

1 cup whole milk yogurt 1 cup Garden greens 3 tbsp MCT oil 1 tbsp flaxseed, ground What you'll need from the store cupboard: 1 cup water 1 packet Stevia, or more to taste

Directions

Add all ingredients in a blender. Blend until smooth and creamy. Serve and enjoy.

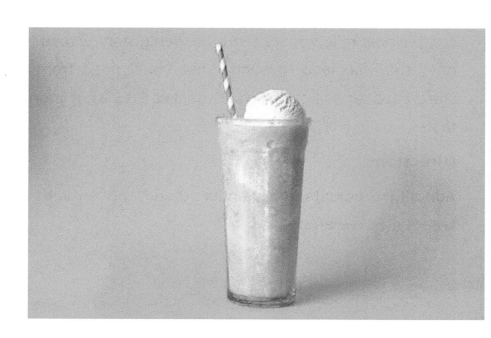

Nutty Arugula Yogurt Smoothie

Preparation time: 5 minutes Cooking time: 0 minutes Servings: 1

Ingredients:

1 cup whole milk yogurt 1 cup baby arugula 3 tbsps avocado oil 2 tbsps macadamia nuts What you'll need from the store cupboard: 1 cup water 1 packet Stevia, or more to taste

Directions

Add all ingredients in a blender. Blend until smooth and creamy. Serve and enjoy.

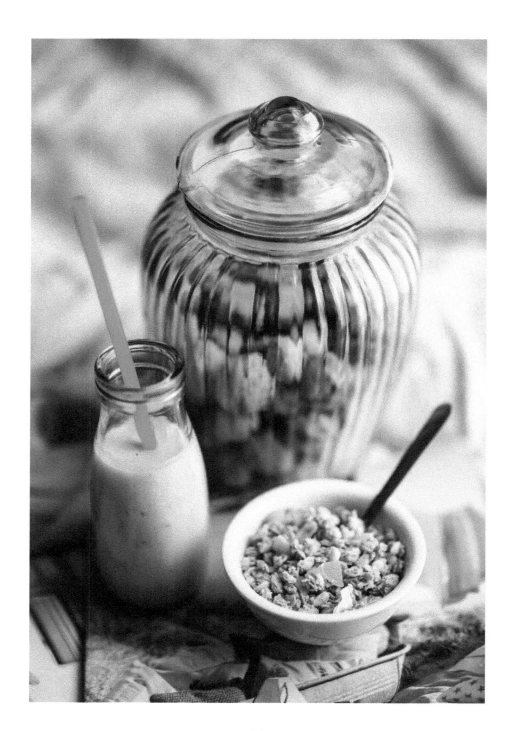

Coffee Flavored Ice Cream

Servings:8 Preparation Time: 1 Hour And 30 Minutes

Ingredients:

1 cup unsweetened almond milk 2 1/2 cups heavy cream divided 1/2 cup powdered erythritol 1 tablespoon coconut oil 1/4 teaspoon xanthan gum 2 tablespoons instant coffee powder 1/2 teaspoon vanilla extract 1/4 teaspoon liquid stevia extract or to taste

Directions

for Cooking: On medium fire, place a saucepan and mix a cup of heavy cream and almond milk. Bring to a boil and then lower fire to a simmer. Frequently stirring, until reduced in half, around an hour and a half. Turn off fire. Whisk in coconut oil ad erythritol until thoroughly combined and smooth. Whisk in liquid stevia extract, vanilla, coffee, and xanthan gum. Let it cool. Meanwhile in a separate bowl, beat on high the remaining cream until stiff. Once the coffee mixture is cooled, fold in whipped cream. Transfer to a lidded container and freeze until solid. Serve and enjoy.

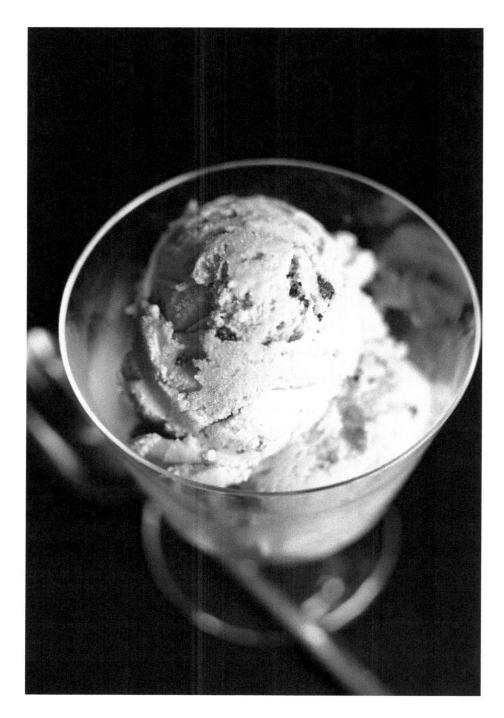

Lava Cake Vegetarian Approved

Servings:1 Preparation Time: 2 Minutes

Ingredients:

2 tbsp cocoa powder 1-2 tbsperythritol 1 medium egg 1 tbsp heavy cream 1/2 tsp vanilla extract 1/4 tsp baking powder 1 pinch salt

Directions

for Cooking: On a small mixing bowl, whisk well cocoa powder and erythritol. In a different bowl, whisk egg until fluffy. Pour into bowl of cocoa and mix well. Stir in vanilla and heavy cream mix well. Add baking powder and salt. Mix well. Lightly grease a ramekin and pour in batter. Stick in the microwave and cook for a minute on high. Let it rest for a minute. Serve and enjoy.

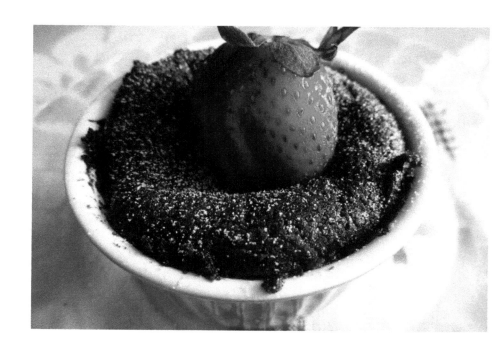

Approved Mud Pie

Servings:10 Preparation Time: 40 Minutes

Ingredients:

1 ½ tsp baking soda 1 cup butter (melted) 1 cup erythritol 1/2 cup cocoa powder (sifted) 1/2 cup heavy cream 1/2 tsp salt 1/4 cup almond milk 2 cups almond flour 2 tbsp coconut flour 2 tsp vanilla extract 3 large eggs Frosting Ingredients: 2 tbsp almond milk 1 1/2 tbsp cocoa powder 1/2 cup powdered erythritol 1/4 cup butter

Directions

for Cooking: Lightly grease a 9x9-inch baking dish with cooking spray and preheat oven to 350oF. In a mixing bowl, whisk well melted butter and eggs. Stir in heavy cream, baking soda, salt, almond milk, ad vanilla extract, Mix thoroughly. Add erythritol, cocoa powder, almond flour, and coconut flour. Mix well. Pour into prepared dish and pop in the oven. Bake for 40 minutes and cool completely. Meanwhile, make the frosting by melting butter in saucepan. Turn off fire and whisk in cocoa powder. Mix well. Add almond milk and powdered erythritol and mix thoroughly until glossy and smooth. Pour frosting on top of cake and refrigerate for at least an hour. Slice into suggested and enjoy.

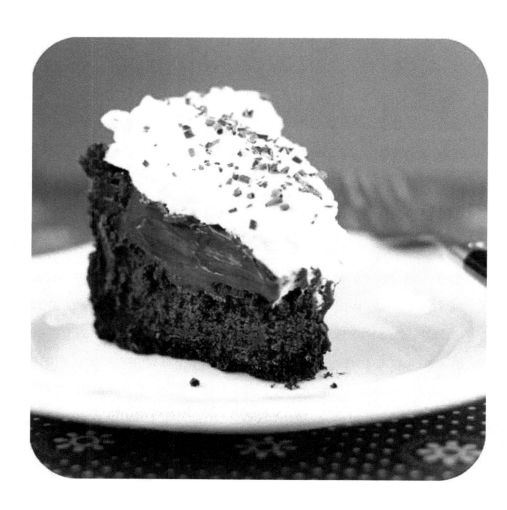

Chocolate Mousse with Avocado

Servings:4 Preparation Time: 10 Minutes

Ingredients:

4 ounces chopped semisweet chocolate 2 large, ripe avocados 3 tablespoons unsweetened cocoa powder 1/4 cup Almond Breeze Unsweetened Almond Milk-Cashew milk Blend 1 teaspoon pure vanilla extract 1/8 teaspoon kosher salt

Directions

for Cooking: In microwave safe bowl, place choco chips and microwave in 15-second interval while mixing every after microwaving until melted. In food processor, add melted chocolate and remaining ingredients and puree until smooth and creamy. Evenly divide into glasses and refrigerate for two hours before serving.

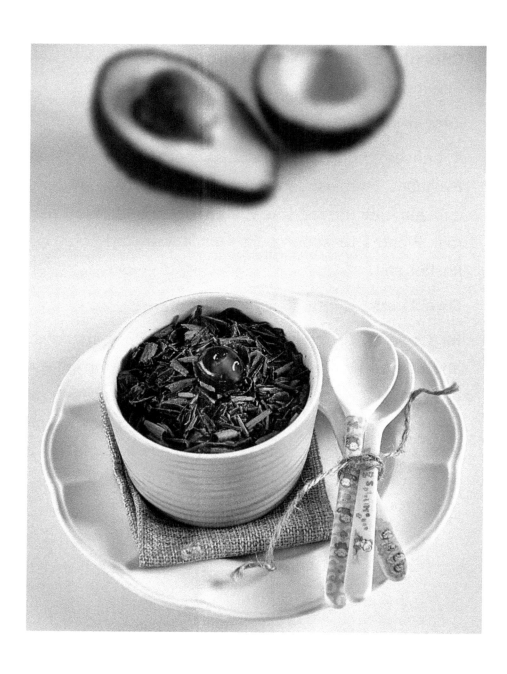

Brownies

Servings: 6 Preparation Time: About 25 Minutes

Ingredients:

1 cup flaxseed meal ¼ cup cocoa powder 1 Tbsp. cinnamon ½ Tbsp. baking powder ½ tsp. salt 1 large egg 2 Tbsp. coconut oil ¼ cup sugar-free caramel syrup ½ cup pumpkin puree 1 tsp. vanilla extract 1 tsp. apple cider vinegar ¼ cup slivered almonds

Directions:

Preheat oven to 350 degrees Fahrenheit Combine all the dry ingredients (flaxseed meal, cocoa powder, cinnamon, baking powder and salt) in aa large mixing bowl and whisk well to combine. In a separate mixing bowl, combine the rest of the ingredients, excluding the almonds. Pour the wet ingredients into the dry ingredients and mix very well with a wooden spoon. Put paper muffin liners in a muffin tin and spoon approximately ¼ cup of batter into each liner. Your Servings should be six muffins. Sprinkle the almonds over the top of the batter, pressing them lightly into the surface so they stick. Bake for about 15 minutes until the batter has risen and is set on top.

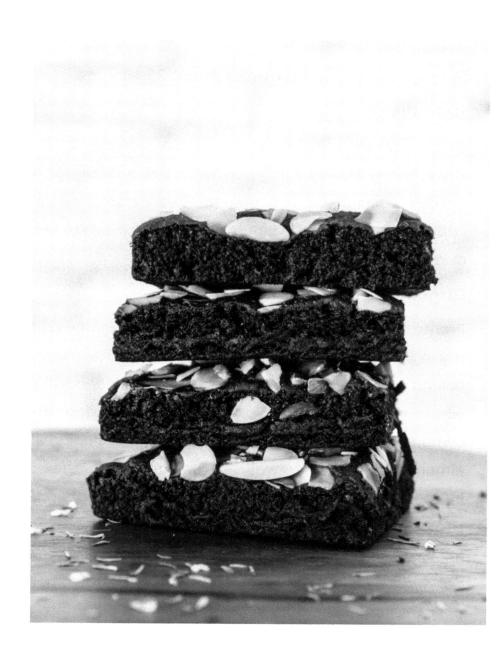

Energizing Ginger Detox Tonic

Servings: 2 Preparation time: 15 minutes

Ingredients:

1/2 teaspoon of grated ginger, fresh 1 small lemon slice 1/8 teaspoon of cayenne pepper 1/8 teaspoon of ground turmeric 1/8 teaspoon of ground cinnamon 1 teaspoon of maple syrup 1 teaspoon of apple cider vinegar 2 cups of boiling water

Directions:

Pour the boiling water into a small saucepan, add and stir the ginger, then let it rest for 8 to 10 minutes, before covering the pan. Pass the mixture through a strainer and into the liquid, add the cayenne pepper, turmeric, cinnamon and stir properly. Add the maple syrup, vinegar, and lemon slice. Add and stir an infused lemon and serve immediately. Warm Spiced

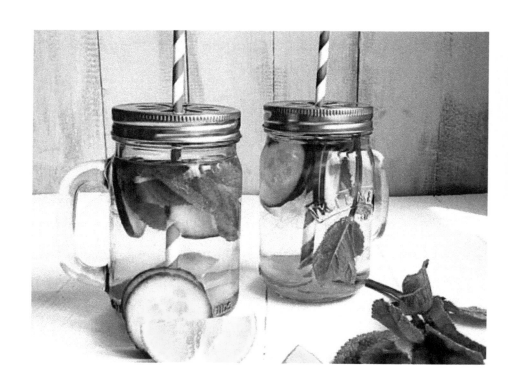

Soothing Ginger Tea Drink

Servings: 8 Preparation time: 2 hours and 15 minutes

Ingredients:

1 tablespoon of minced gingerroot 2 tablespoons of honey 15 green tea bags 32 fluid ounce of white grape juice 2 quarts of boiling water

Directions:

Pour water into a 4-quarts slow cooker, immerse tea bags, cover the cooker and let stand for 10 minutes. After 10 minutes, remove and discard tea bags and stir in remaining ingredients. Return cover to slow cooker, then plug in and let cook at high heat setting for 2 hours or until heated through. When done, strain the liquid and serve hot or cold.

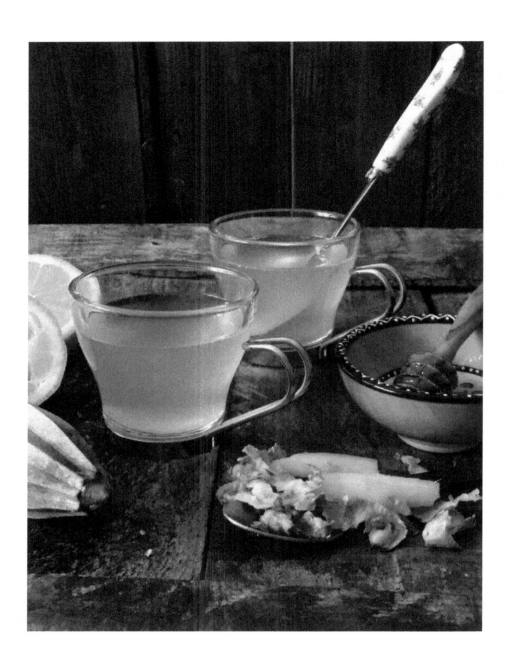

Lightning Source UK Ltd.
Milton Keynes UK
UKHW020809250521
384334UK00001B/107

9 781802 697261